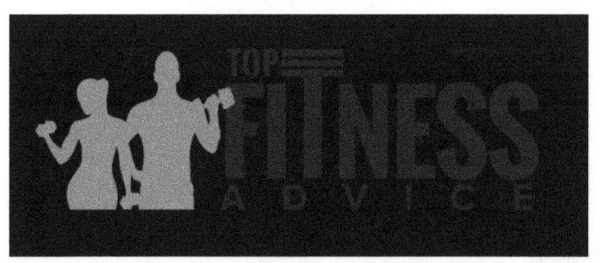

DIET

The Quick & Easy Guide To Healthy Eating So You Lose Weight, Look Good & Feel Great! (BONUS: Comprehensive Shopping List Included)

Sarah Talene

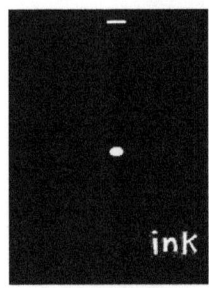

First published in 2017 by Venture Ink Publishing

Copyright © Top Fitness Advice 2019

All rights reserved.

No part of this book may be reproduced in any form without permission in writing from the author. No part of this publication may be reproduced or transmitted in any form or by any means, mechanic, electronic, photocopying, recording, by any storage or retrieval system, or transmitted by email without the permission in writing from the author and publisher.

Requests to the publisher for permission should be addressed to
publishing@ventureink.co

For more information about the contents of this book or questions to the author, please contact Sarah Talene at
sarah@topfitnessadvice.com

Disclaimer

This book provides wellness management information in an informative and educational manner only, with information that is general in nature and that is not specific to you, the reader. The contents of this book are intended to assist you and other readers in your personal wellness efforts. Consult your physician regarding the applicability of any information provided in this book to you.

Nothing in this book should be construed as personal advice or diagnosis, and must not be used in this manner. The information provided about conditions is general in nature. This information does not cover all possible uses, actions, precautions, side-effects, or interactions of medicines, or medical procedures. The information in this book should not be considered as complete and does not cover all diseases, ailments, physical conditions, or their treatment.

You should consult with your physician before beginning any exercise, weight loss, or health care program. This book should not be used in place of a call or visit to a competent health-care professional. You should consult a health care professional before adopting any of the suggestions in this book or before drawing inferences from it.

Any decision regarding treatment and medication for your condition should be made with the advice and consultation of a qualified health care professional. If you have, or suspect you have, a health-care problem, then you should immediately contact a qualified health care professional for treatment.

No Warranties: The author and publisher don't guarantee or warrant the quality, accuracy, completeness, timeliness, appropriateness or suitability of the information in this book, or of any product or services referenced in this book.

The information in this book is provided on an "as is" basis and the author and publisher make no representations or warranties of any kind with respect to this information. This book may contain inaccuracies, typographical errors, or other errors.

Liability Disclaimer: The publisher, author, and other parties involved in the creation, production, provision of information, or delivery of this book specifically disclaim any responsibility, and shall not be held liable for any damages, claims, injuries, losses, liabilities, costs, or obligations including any direct, indirect, special, incidental, or consequences damages (collectively known as "Damages") whatsoever and howsoever caused, arising out of, or in connection with the use or misuse of the site and the information contained within it, whether such Damages arise in contract, tort, negligence, equity, statute law, or by way of other legal theory.

Table of Contents

Disclaimer	3
Who is this book for?	7
What will this book teach you?	9
Introduction	11
The 7 Steps to Healthy Eating	17
Ready-to-Go Shopping List	23
7 Ways to Stay Healthy When Eating Out	27
7-Day Menu Plan	29
How to Boost Your Metabolism	33
36 Fat Burning Super Foods	45
20 Tasty Super Food Smoothies and Soup Recipes	59
8 Reasons Why You Are Not Losing Body Fat	85
Conclusion	95
Final Words	97

Would you prefer to listen to my book, rather than read it?

Download the audiobook version for free!

If you go to the special link below and sign up to Audible as a new customer, you can get the audiobook version of my book completely free.

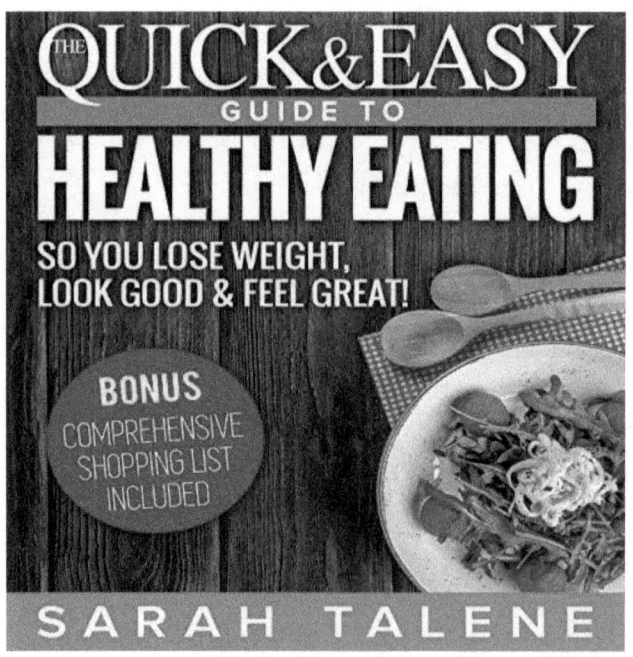

Go here to get your audiobook version for free:

TopFitnessAdvice.com/go/Diet

Who is this book for?

Are you sick and tired of always being tired?

Is channel-surfing the only exercise you have the energy to do when you get home?

If you want to make a change, you need to ensure that you give your body the nutrition that it needs.

But do you know where to start?

There is so much conflicting advice out there that it is tough to know who is right.

Some people tell you that carbs are the bad guys. Others say that too much protein is bad for you.

Who do you listen to?

If you are looking for a simple, clean eating plan and don't have the time to wade through mountains of advice, this book is for you.

The plan laid out is simple to follow and provides ample nutrition to fuel your new lifestyle.

Do you want to have boundless energy?

Do you want to look great and feel great?

Are you tired of diets that leave you starving, physically and emotionally?

Do you want to find out why your current eating plan is not working for you?

What will this book teach you?

The principles of healthy eating are quite simple, but all the conflicting advice can be confusing.

This book will teach you how you can start to eat meals that are healthy and nutritious.

You will learn how to eat more healthily in your daily life – whether you are at home or going out with friends.

This is a whole new way of looking at nutrition – instead of focusing solely on calorie content, you are going to be taught to look for foods that give you the most bang for your buck.

The book lays it out simply for you – there is even a 7-day sample plan to get you started. But it doesn't stop there. You will also learn how to supercharge your metabolism and what foods will help you to torch fat.

In addition, you will learn what power foods to eat to flush out the toxins and really rev up your energy levels. The recipes at the end of the book taste great and help make healthy eating a lot more fun.

Your body is a finely built machine.

This book will teach you how to keep it tuned for optimal performance. You will learn not only how you should be eating but also what mistakes can derail your weight loss efforts.

Get yourself out of the slow lane and start living the life you were meant to.

Introduction

The term "healthy eating" covers a broad range of subjects.

At the moment, it is also quite a controversial term. The only thing that the experts seem to agree on is that they disagree about what "healthy eating" consists of.

Now, that's all good and well but it doesn't help you out if you want to learn how to supercharge your nutrition.

If you really want to get your body firing on all cylinders, you need the right nutrition information and you need it now. And you don't want to have to sort through all the confusing data out there.

Not to worry – I have done that for you. I have laid out a simple plan that is proven to be effective.

With my experience in the field of physical fitness, I have zeroed in on what works when you need to perform at a higher level.

And it's not all about starving yourself or eating foods that you really cannot stand.

It's not about isolating yourself from your friends for fear of a few bites of junk food.

What it is about is making the right food choices. And with this book, this will be easy for you.

I've made it as simple as possible. I give you lists of foods that you should concentrate on. I've scrapped calorie counting – it's not effective anyway – and concentrated on giving you food that is naturally nutritious and wholesome. This plan will help you relearn how to trust your own body and its natural hunger signals.

You have a 7-day meal plan to get you started.

Want to take it up a notch? Read about the power foods that boost your health and energy levels.

Learn which foods to eat to boost your body's own fat-blasting systems. The basic plan is simple, the recipes provided taste great.

Are you ready to turn your body into a lean, mean, fat-blasting machine?

Weight Loss is HARD!

Discover How to Make It EASIER to Lose Weight & Keep It OFF Forever (This Is The ONLY Book You NEED to Read)

For this month only, you can get Sarah's best-selling & most popular guide absolutely free – *The #1 Weight Loss Guide*.

Get Your FREE Copy Here:
TopFitnessAdvice.com/Freebie

It's time to stop struggling with your weight loss efforts that don't seem to work.

Discover how you can start seeing real results by next week (without changing much in your life). With this guide, readers were able to significantly improve their weight loss results. So, it's highly recommended that you get this guide, especially while it's free!

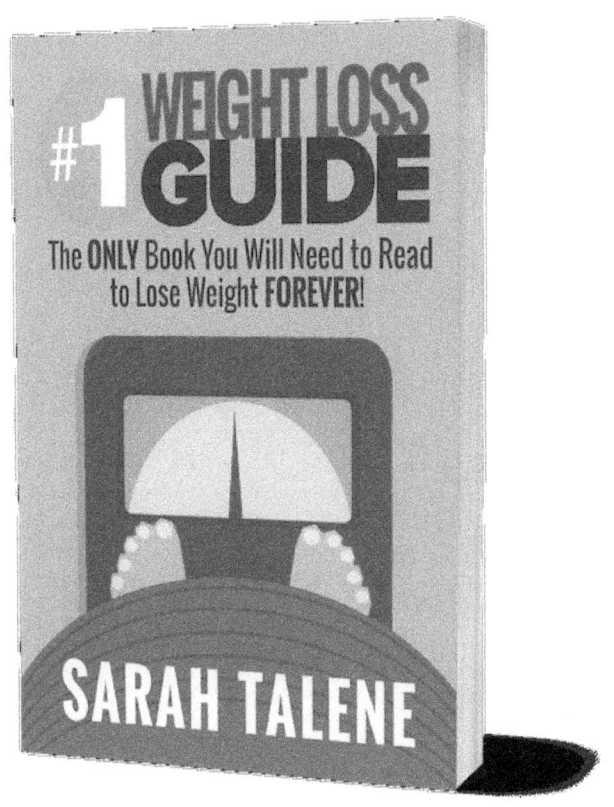

Get Your FREE Copy Here:
TopFitnessAdvice.com/Freebie

The 7 Steps to Healthy Eating

Fat loss begins in the kitchen and the key to any workout program is healthy nutrition.

I come across many clients who work long hours who claim they honestly don't have the energy to exercise after a hard day at the office. The solution is simple; a clean eating plan that focuses on natural foods.

Not only will your energy levels improve your skin will look and feel better, you'll feel less fatigued in the afternoons and you will also sleep well.

1. **Week 1:** Eat as much white meat, fish, vegetables and fruit as you want, except bananas. Aim to eat more vegetables than fruit as fruit contains a lot of sugar.

   Have a fist full of nuts and seeds a day (milled flax seeds are a good choice). You can have eggs, herbal tea and coconut water. You may also have corn, sweet potato and other root vegetables but **not** potatoes

   No dairy, alcohol, refined carbohydrates (read below), sugar, red meat, caffeine or packaged foods. (It sounds harsh but you'll survive!)

2. **Week 2 and 3:** As above but you can add in a fistful of carbohydrates on Monday, Wednesday and Friday.

This should follow on from your hardest HIIT workout routines.

Choose from this list **ONLY**:

- Brown Rice
- Oats
- Quinoa
- Cous Cous

3. **Eliminate these foods from your life:**

   - **Dairy** - Just for the first week. You will get all your calcium from green vegetables. If you are concerned about adequate amounts, try a supplement as well but this is not compulsory.

   - **Caffeine** - (except green tea) Caffeine increases the effects of cortisol and actually stores fat around your middle. Replace with herbal teas such as Liquorice tea which is great for stabilizing a sweet tooth and mint tea which can calm discomfort during digestion.

   - **Refined carbohydrates** - White pasta, biscuits, chocolates, bread, noodles, cereal, crackers (or anything that contains wheat)

   - **Processed sugar** - Anything with syrup or sweetener and anything ending in 'ose'. Avoid artificial sweeteners.

- **Ready meals** - and prepackaged meals. These are very high in salt and empty calories. Everything should be fresh and natural.

4. **Drink plenty of water.**

All chemical reactions in the body take place in water including calorie burning.

Dehydration causes the body to fatigue and reduces the capacity for fat reduction; it will also decrease concentration, efficiency and increases the effects of ageing.

Drink a pint of cold water every morning and half an hour before lunch and dinner and aim for at least 6 glasses a day.

Once you feel thirsty you are already dehydrated. Place a reminder on your phone to go off at regular intervals to remind you to grab a drink and keep a bottle of water in your bag or at your desk.

5. **Include at every meal:**

Protein - Portion size about a hand span worth

- Lean chicken, turkey, duck, quorn
- Free range eggs
- Fish: Tuna, smoked mackerel, kippers, salmon, prawns, mussels, squid, halibut (pretty much any white fish)

- Raw nuts: Walnuts, Brazils, almonds, macadamia nuts, pecans, flax seeds, sesame seeds, pumpkin and sunflower seeds.
- Beans and lentils
- Raw nut butters

Fat sources

- Extra virgin olive oil
- Fish oil
- Cod liver oil (supplement or liquid)
- Flax seeds
- Avocadoes
- Coconut oil
- Raw nuts

Fibrous Carbohydrates - Portion 2/3 of your plate should be green vegetables

- All vegetables
- All fruits

6. **Eat little and often.**

Including a mid-morning and mid-afternoon snack. This will ensure your metabolism keeps ticking over and avoids that 4pm slump.

Try one of these options:

- Oat cakes and cottage cheese
- A piece of fruit

- Vegetable crudités and hummus
- A handful of nuts or seeds
- Fruit Smoothie
- Tbsp. of natural yogurt with berries and Agave nectar

7. **Don't count calories.**

This is a favorite of mine when taking on new clients who have been steadily following 1000 calories a day plan and not losing any weight.

Calories are subjective and your body will respond in different ways depending on where the calories are coming from. A 600-calorie meal consisting of vegetables and proteins will be broken down slowly and converted into glycogen for use as energy leaving you fuller for longer.

A 600-calorie meal; obtained through a slice of pizza or a chocolate cake will be broken down quickly and contains empty calories that the body cannot convert or use but will instead instantly be stored as fat leaving you hungry and with slightly fuller fat cells.

When following an exercise plan such as "The 5-Minute Workout" you may need more calories to keep the fire burning in order to lose more fat.

Ready-to-Go Shopping List

Choose foods from each section. You need to have protein and vegetables at each meal.

Complex carbohydrates are only for post workout meals.

Fruit

- Apples
- Blueberries
- Plums
- Strawberries
- Cherries
- Mangoes
- Clementine's
- Watermelons
- Lemons
- Pears
- Bananas
- Raspberries
- Melons

Vegetables

- Tomatoes
- Red onions
- Cucumbers
- Peas
- Bamboo shoots

- Kidney beans
- Broccoli
- Cauliflower
- Garlic
- Avocadoes
- Pepper
- Celery
- Tomatoes
- Sweet corn
- Broad beans
- Green beans
- Cabbage
- Celeriac
- Asparagus
- Courgettes
- Mushrooms
- Squash
- Leeks
- Spinach
- Carrots
- Onions
- Chicory
- Rocket

Dressings

- Olive oil
- Balsamic vinegar
- Chili oil
- Hummus

- Agave nectar
- Apple cider vinegar
- Lemon juice

Complex carbohydrates (post workout)

- Cous cous
- Quinoa
- Brown rice

Complex carbohydrates (allowed)

- Oatcakes

Fresh fish/meat/soya

- Tuna
- Prawns
- Salmon
- Any white fish
- Lean chicken
- Lean turkey
- Tofu
- Quorn

Dairy

- Eggs
- Natural Yogurt

Teas

- Green tea
- Chamomile
- Liquorice
- Mint
- Sage
- Nettle
- Echinacea
- Tulsi

I hope that you are enjoying this book so far, and if you could spare 30 seconds, I would greatly appreciate you leaving a review on Amazon.com.

7 Ways to Stay Healthy When Eating Out

In the corporate world, it is very common to eat out on a regular basis and I also have clients who simply cannot be bothered to cook after a long day at the office and will eat take out at least two or three times a week. It is important to make healthy choices when eating out this often as rich food combined with big restaurant portions can play havoc with your waistline.

Restaurants

1. If drinking wine, have a glass of water between each glass to fill you up.

2. Try to avoid eating the bread rolls whilst waiting for your dinner to be served, ask for a small side salad instead.

3. Once your meal is served eat a portion of protein which is approximately the size of your hand with double the amount in vegetables and if you want to have a dessert, then don't eat any complex carbohydrates with your main course.

Takeaway

1. At Chinese restaurants avoid deep fried items such as spring rolls/ fried noodles/ crispy meats and sweet and sour items and try boiled rather than fried rice.

2. At Indian restaurants avoid Kormas, creamy sauces or anything fried or dipped in butter. Tikka, Tandoori, Pilau rice and Naan bread without butter are better choices.

Fast Food

1. Burgers tend to be lower in fat than chicken fish sandwiches, but order burgers without mayonnaise or sauce and avoid extra cheese as this significantly increases the fat content.

2. Go for salad instead of chips as a side option.

7-Day Menu Plan

❖ Day 1

- **Breakfast** - Plain natural yogurt and fresh berries (if you need a sweet kick add some agave nectar)

- **Lunch** - Mixed green salad with tuna and quinoa (This can be cooked veg as well!)

- **Dinner** - Roasted vegetables (broccoli / carrots / garlic / peppers / cauliflower / courgettes / baby sweet corn) with lean piece of chicken and mashed butterbeans.

❖ Day 2

- **Breakfast** - Boiled egg with rye bread and a piece of fresh fruit.

- **Lunch** - Mixed bean and veg soup (Covent Garden soup / Tesco veg soup) and a piece of fruit.

- **Dinner** - Brown rice with chicken, onions and garlic fried with peppers, green beans and tomatoes

❖ Day 3

- **Breakfast** - Fresh berries with natural yogurt (agave nectar if necessary)

- **Lunch** - Beetroot and green leaves with sunflower and pumpkin seeds and handful of prawns. Fruit smoothie for after (Handful of Raspberries, 1 apple, 1 banana, 1 orange and as much spinach and kale as you can squeeze in. Add apple juice for consistency)

- **Dinner** - Fillet of fish (unbattered!) with spinach and asparagus sprinkled with lemon and cupful of brown rice.

❖ **Day 4**

- **Breakfast** - rye bread with marmite, boiled egg and piece of fruit.

- **Lunch** - Green salad with chicken strips, avocado and Clementine pieces. Fruit smoothie as above.

- **Dinner** - Mushroom stir fry (beansprouts / carrots / onions / garlic / chili / asparagus / mushrooms / green beans / mange tout / baby sweet corn) with king prawns and butterbean mash.

❖ **Day 5**

- **Breakfast** - Cottage cheese on oat cakes with piece of fresh fruit and handful of walnuts.

- **Lunch** - Green soup and oat cakes (In a pan fry 1 onion, 1 stick of celery and garlic with extra virgin olive oil till brown. Add 1 litre of veg stock, 1 courgette, 1 bunch of broccoli, 250g of asparagus,

250g of green beans, and 180g of spinach and bring to boil. Blend to create smooth soup) takes 15 minutes.

- **Dinner** - Oven cooked salmon with steamed veg (broccoli / asparagus / spinach / carrots).

❖ Day 6

- **Breakfast** - Berry compote (blueberries / raspberries / strawberries and red berries with natural plain yogurt)

- **Lunch** - Balsamic chicken salad (Green beans / roasted peppers / tomatoes / boneless, skinless chicken breast and balsamic vinegar)

- **Dinner** - Tomatoes minestrone soup. Carrot, celery and apple salad with sliced grilled chicken and natural yogurt.

❖ Day 7

Cheat day!

Having a cheat day once a week will stop you feeling so deprived and allow you to treat yourself within reason.

Treat yourself to a slice of cake or a couple of pieces of pizza but don't go overboard. The sudden shock of extra glucose in the body will help to regenerate the metabolism and stop the body reaching a plateau. This is due to the release of hormones.

Leptin is a hormone which controls many metabolic processes in your body and it is also responsible for fat loss. The more leptin you have the faster you lose fat. The silly thing is the more fat you lose the lower your leptin levels which is why it is so hard to lose the last few lbs.

Leptin is produced in fat cells so the smaller you are and the fewer fat cells, the less leptin you'll produce.

When you restrict calories, you reduce leptin.

Despite what you may think we are not trying to restrict calories on this plan, however I am not asking you to reduce calories I am just encouraging you to get them from cleaner, higher energy foods. Whilst doing this if we constantly regulate our leptin levels fat loss will be quicker.

This is where cheat days come in. When you eat the foods that are high in extra calories that your body doesn't need you will increase the amount of leptin produced in fat cells and kick start that fat burning furnace for another week!

Once again, thank you for reading this book, and I hope you're getting a lot of valuable information. I would greatly appreciate it if you could take 30 seconds to leave me a review for this book on Amazon.com.

How to Boost Your Metabolism

To help burn off calories faster, you need to give your metabolism a good kick-start.

- **Drink Water**

    Water increases your metabolism significantly. Research has shown that, after drinking a 16-oz. cup of water, people were burning off more calories. On top of that, 30 minutes after drinking the water, they were still burning up to 30% more calories than those who didn't drink it.

- **Eat First, Sweat Later**

    To lose weight you have to eat less calories than you are burning but this does not mean starving yourself. You need to eat the right foods to lose that fat and, to digest the food and storm the nutrients in it, your body requires energy.

    If you exercise before you eat, you've used up your energy stores and your food won't digest properly. Eat a good meal, full of proteins and good carbs before you exercise to boost your metabolic burn rate.

- **Eat Again**

    Instead of eating one or two meals a day, divide your allowance into three good meals and two snacks. Eating smaller and more regular meals is better for you than sticking to two or three main meals and leads to for more efficient fat burning.

- **Eat Plenty of Protein**

    Protein is the part of your meal that makes you feel fuller for longer. As well as that, your body will use up more calories when it digests protein than it does when it has to break down fat or carbohydrates. Eat plenty of eggs, lean meats, seafood, poultry and dairy, along with avocado to raise the leucine levels in your body – this is a required amino acid for maintaining your muscle bulk and for burning off calories.

- **Caffeine Isn't All Bad**

    200 mg of caffeine per day is a safe level to drink and it will make you less likely to store fat. This is because, at the right levels, it stimulates the body to use fat, especially when you are exercising.

Everyone wants to feel good, to feel alert, rested and full of energy but, for most, this is just a dream. The reality is we live in a harsh world, where time is in short supply and stress is in abundance. Lack of sleep combined with poor diet and stress leads to illness and exhaustion.

Fatigue is one of the worst things for the human body; it breaks us down emotionally and physically and it wreaks total havoc on our immune systems, which opens the way for chronic disease.

But, we all have the power needed to make that change, to give our bodies the energy boost they need and to feel fantastic with it.

Regular exercise, learning how to manage stress and sleeping properly are all critical factors in being able to combat fatigue but you can also make a change to your eating habits.

The following are ten ways in which you can use the food you eat to give you energy that lasts throughout the day.

1. Eat Foods that are Dense in Nutrients

The best way to boost your metabolism to convert your food into energy is eat foods that contain the right minerals and vitamins – and plenty of them.

If you eat the right food, all the cells in your body will produce energy to keep you going.

2. Eat Foods that are High in Antioxidants

These are the scavengers that clean out all the chemicals and toxins in the body that are wearing you down. Eat plenty of fruits and vegetables and other plant-based foods rather than taking them in supplement form.

Eating too much of some nutrients can be risky so get around this by eating only whole foods, like colorful berries, melons and dark green leafy vegetables.

3. Eating your Omega-3's

Over the years, research has shown that plenty of omega-3 in your diet can improve your memory, mood and thinking, all of which are closely related to energy. Try to eat one good helping per day in the form of flax oil or seeds, fish, hemp oil or seeds, leafy greens and walnuts.

4. Stop Dieting

Most diets are no good for the human body because they require you to deprive your body of certain foods. You should not cut your calories down too much because this just decreases your metabolism. That is why many people who are on strict diets often complain of lethargy.

And, as your metabolism slows down, your body will burn off less calories, which means the ultimate result, is a gain in weight. Eat the right amount of calorie needs every day and eat them in the right foods, combined with regular exercise if you want to successfully drop the pounds.

5. Don't Skip Breakfast

Yes, it is so easy, when you are running late and there are those who think that to lose weight they have to skip a meal. It is the wrong meal to skip. Breakfast is the most important meal of the day as it gets your metabolism off and running and a good breakfast will keep your energy levels up until it's time for lunch.

Instead of hitting the bagel bar or eating stodgy cereals, go for eggs, fresh fruit, whole grain cereal and nuts.

6. Don't Pass on Snacks

It is important to eat enough of the right foods to keep you blood glucose levels steady throughout the day, and that will keep your energy levels steady as well. Snack on dried fruit and nuts, yoghurt with granola, whole grain crackers, fresh raw vegetables and fruits.

7. Drink Your Fluids

Hydration is an important part of weight loss and of keeping your energy levels high. Your body needs a lot of water to function at its best but, unless you are doing endurance training, skip the energy drinks and vitamin waters.

Instead, drink plain water or water with fresh fruit chunks in it and aim to drink at least one cup every couple of hours.

8. Be a Designated Driver

That will help you to cut out one of the biggest enemies of those who want to lose weight – alcohol. As well as acting as a depressant, alcohol can also act as a stimulant, interrupting your sleep patterns and causing tiredness the following day.

If you are relying on a drink every night to help you fall asleep, you are doing the wrong thing. Cutting out the alcohol will help you to sleep better.

If you do want to have a drink occasionally, stick to red wine. It is an antioxidant but do be aware that you cannot drink if you are on certain medications, have high blood pressure or anxiety.

9. Caffeine – Little or None

Caffeine should be used carefully and in small amounts. Although it seems as if it is giving you an energy boost, it won't last for long and you will know it when it wears off.

And never use caffeine as a meal replacement! Green tea is a better choice of caffeine as it also contains antioxidants and theanine, which is an essential amino acid that helps you to stay calm.

10. Eat Power Foods

Try to stick to nutritional foods that provide energy, a list of 10 are below. Later on, I will go into more details on foods to eat to help you burn off fat.

- Nuts, especially almonds
- Avocado
- Dark leafy greens, such as watercress, kale, spinach, collard or beet greens
- Whole grains that are intact, like quinoa, millet, brown rice or amaranth

- Ground flax seeds
- White beans, lentils, black beans
- Dried fruits such as dates but in moderation
- Berries – blackberries, strawberries, raspberries, blueberries, etc.
- Sea vegetables such as Nori, hijiki, dulse, etc.
- Edamame – whole young soy beans

Herbs and spices are a fantastic way of giving otherwise bland food a taste boost and using them is one of the best ways to enjoy nutritious foods that may not taste so great.

Not many people know that herbs and spices are full of health benefits. The following are ten of the best to boost your health and excite your taste buds.

1. Cayenne Pepper

Adds a dash of spice and also helps to enhance bodily functions. Cayenne helps to boost the metabolism, in turn increasing the amount of fat that your body burns off and it improves your blood flow.

This means that the essential nutrients and vitamins in your food are moved through the body far more efficiently, allowing your body to function better.

2. Black Pepper

Similar to cayenne, black pepper helps to boost the metabolism and it helps to improve the digestive process, which in turn helps the body to shed weight. It also contains anti-cancer properties.

3. Ginger

Ginger is good for suppressing the appetite and aiding digestion. It also works to warm up the body, increasing metabolism and helping more calories to burn off. Ginger is good for shifting toxins out of the body, in particular out of the fat cells.

4. Ginseng

Ginseng helps to boost metabolism and raise energy levels and is popular in energy drinks. It is a great one to use just before you do short high intensity workouts.

5. Chamomile Tea

Chamomile tea is great for relaxation and helps to reduce stress levels. It also helps to stop emotional eating in the evenings, thus preventing weight gain and it helps you to sleep better.

Chamomile contains anti-inflammatory properties, helping to reduce the inflammation that causes so many different diseases, and it is high in antioxidants, eliminating free radicals from the body.

6. Cumin

Cumin tends to be mixed with other spices to give a nice flavor to Mexican, Indian, Middle Eastern and Mediterranean foods.

It is used as a part of Ayurvedic medicine, helps to boost your immune system, decrease your cholesterol and contains anti-oxidant properties. It helps to increase the energy levels, allowing for more calories to be burned off.

7. Turmeric

Turmeric is fantastic for people who crave junk food. It helps to boost the function of the liver and to balance out hormones, which also prevents binges. It is a powerful antioxidant that helps to maintain good joints and skin, as well as vision.

It works to enhance the immune system, digestive processes and the function of the liver as well as stabilizing blood glucose levels and cutting down on the amount of fat storage.

8. Cinnamon

This is a sweet spice that helps to boost metabolism and improve insulin sensitivity, thus helping to boost fat burning and control the blood sugar levels.

9. Mustard

Mustard helps to boost weight loss because it is full of B-complex vitamins, such as niacin, folates, riboflavin and thiamine, all of which increase the metabolism. One teaspoon of mustard can help to boost metabolism by 25%.

Mustard is also high in magnesium and selenium which provides anti-inflammatory properties to help fight off disease. It is also a good source of zeaxanthins, carotenes and luteins, all of which are good antioxidants that help to eliminate free radicals.

10. Cardamom

This is a sweet spice that is used in Indian cooking and it helps to promote a healthy digestion and increases your metabolism.

It is a commonly used ingredient in Ayurvedic medicine and has been shown to help mouth ulcers, high blood pressure, and depression. It has both anti-oxidative and anti-inflammatory properties and can also help to slow down the aging process.

So, the next time you are preparing your meals, add in one or more of these herbs and spices. Not only will your food taste nicer, your health will be better and your metabolism will be faster, helping you to burn off fat more efficiently.

Enjoying this book?

Check out my other best sellers!

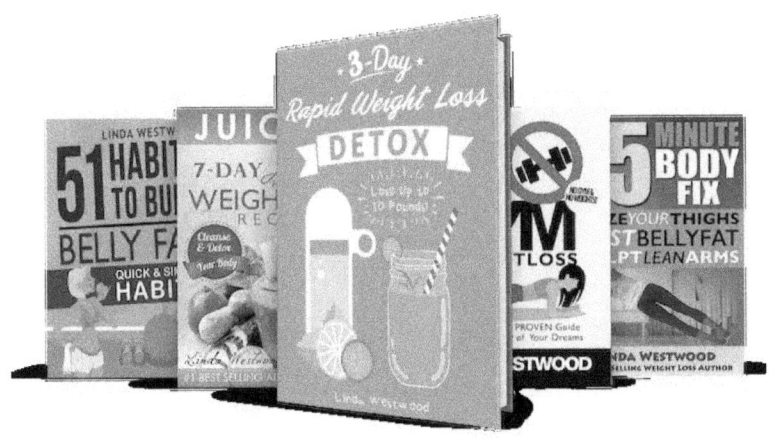

Get your next book on sale here:

TopFitnessAdvice.com/go/books

36 Fat Burning Super Foods

Food is not our enemy but so many diets will have you believe that it is. You don't need to eat a diet that is lacking in taste or looks to lose weight and you certainly do not need to deprive yourself just because the latest fad diet says you mustn't at certain foods.

The following 36 foods are super foods that will help you to burn off fat more efficiently. However, don't get stuck on just one of them; introduce a few of them at a time to your weekly menu and, as time goes on, you will find that you are eating more and more of them.

- **Tomatoes**

    Who really cares if a tomato is a fruit or a vegetable? All that is important is knowing that a tomato contains loads of goodness that can help your body in the long terms and, over the short term, it can help you to lose some weight.

    They are low in calories but contain enough fiber to keep you regular and make you feel fuller. Tomatoes contain lycopene as well, which are antioxidants, helpful in removing free radicals and other toxins from your system.

- **Oranges**

Oranges are full of vitamin C, which is needed to keep your body functioning at an optimal level. However, many people avoid oranges when they are trying to burn fat because they are worried about the sugar level.

Oranges do contain sugar and, if you eat too many of them and don't burn off the sugar, it can turn to fat. However, they are low in calories and high in fiber, which helps keep your glucose levels regular. To help you to lose weight, moderate how much you eat and use it as a way of curbing a craving for candy.

- **Oats**

Oats contain fiber, which helps to boost the metabolism, although many of those who do diets like Atkins and Paleo would disagree. A bowl of oatmeal is a fabulous way to start off the day. It isn't just full of fiber; it also contains anti-oxidants and lots of other minerals. Oats are a good way of cutting cholesterol levels.

- **Spices**

You do not need to eat bland tasteless food when you are trying to shed some pounds so get experimenting with the contents of your spice rack. Some of them contain thermo genic properties, which help to boost the metabolism, and all of them give dishes a great taste.

Mustard seed goes great on an entrée and will boost your metabolism while ginger helps your digestive system.

Ginseng boosts energy and black pepper can help you to burn off calories. Turmeric is good for breaking up fat.

- **Sweet Potatoes**

These are a fantastic addition to a diet, as a replacement for normal potatoes because they contain fewer calories and can help you to feel fuller for longer. Sweet potatoes are also loaded with potassium, fiber, vitamin B6 and vitamin C, making them the perfect replacement for a food that is normally shunned by dieters everywhere.

- **Apples**

Not many people realize just how good an apple is. They are sweet enough to be a good replacement for sweet cravings and you can easily see why they end up in desserts. They are also low in calories, low in fat and low in sodium while being high in fiber.

The fiber fills you up for longer and stops you from eating in between meals, and they also help with your digestive system too. Make sure you chew and apple thoroughly to get the best out of it.

- **Nuts**

Every diet plan in the world include nuts and they are the one food that unites the vegetarians with the meat loving paleo dieters. They come straight from the earth and a small handful of nuts, raw and organic ones like pecans, walnuts or almonds, can be a tasty and filling snack that keep soya going for a few hours. You can also chop them and add them to a salad or sprinkle them over your food. Nuts are full of good healthy fats and full of flavor.

- **Quinoa**

Quinoa is just starting to become popular in mainstream diets and the weight loss normally happens when you switch out rice or potatoes, or other starchy sides with quinoa. You get the full benefits of a well-rounded meals with all the vitamins contained in the quinoa. It is low in calories, low GI and full of taste.

- **Beans**

Beans are a staple part of many diets and should be included as part of your weekly menu. They help to regulate glucose levels, help with digestion because of their high fiber content and are a great replacement for high carb foods.

Black beans are particularly good for snacking on and you will find that many restaurants provide them as an alternative to bread.

- **Egg Whites**

The egg debate is an age-old one. Some people say the yolks are fine to eat, others say not, that you should only eat egg white. Whole eggs are a fantastic source of protein and the biggest debate rages around the cholesterol and fat levels in the yolks. If you want to be safe, eat the whites on and start adding yolks back in at a later date.

- **Grapefruit**

Grapefruits are an excellent fat burning food and this is being proved with more research every year. Grapefruit helps to kick start the digestive system, making fat burning an easier and more efficient process. You can start with pure grapefruit juice if you want and work your way up to eating a grapefruit.

- **Chicken Breast**

Chicken breast is a staple part of many diets, although it is obviously no good if you are going vegetarian or vegan. It is low in fat and high in protein and is far healthier to eat than the dark meat from a chicken.

Do remember to take the skin off, as this is where all the fat is and use a variety of spices and herbs to boost the flavor. Combine eating chicken breast with strength training to help tone up your muscles, which will boost your metabolism rate as well.

- **Bananas**

Bananas are one of the most natural foods to eat and are the subject of many research programs for their effect on weight loss. They are so easy to add in to your diet on a daily basis because they are such a versatile fruit. They can be eaten on their own, chopped up and added to oatmeal or yoghurt and are a great source of potassium, natural sugar and energy.

- **Pears**

Pears are often dismissed from a diet but they really should be included. They are full of flavor, and contain a whole range of benefits, which are great for weight loss.

They help you to feel fuller for longer and they are different in consistency to apples and other fruits, which makes their fiber content more effective than others are. They can be eaten as they are, chopped up or cooked.

- **Pine Nuts**

Pine nuts include a phytonutrient that can help to suppress the appetite, which means you can ditch the cost of buying expensive diet pills that are full of chemicals to do the same thing.

They are tiny and they are crunchy so you can eat a lot without worrying about the effect of them and without ruining your weight loss efforts. These are one food you can binge on without any trouble.

- **Mushrooms**

You won't see the benefits if you switch pepperoni for mushrooms on your next pizza but if you start increasing the amount you are eating, along with a range of other healthier foods, you will see a difference, because they are low in calories and high in vitamins.

Don't be boring though; try all different ones from the supermarket and enjoy a range of textures, flavors and other great benefits.

- **Lentils**

    Lentils are another food that is gaining in popularity and are not just for a vegetarian diet. They contain fiber, which helps your digestive system keep your blood sugar from spiking and help you to feel fuller for longer.

    They are also full of protein and help to keep cholesterol levels down as well as helping the body to process carbohydrates better.

- **Hot Peppers**

    Jalapenos, chipotles and habaneros peppers are excellent weight loss foods while adding a healthy kick to the flavor of a dish.

    Instead of ruining your stomach lining like some believe, these will actually help to protect your stomach and prevent ulcers by killing off the bad bacteria.

- **Broccoli**

    Broccoli is one of the best superfoods. Not only are they full of anti-oxidants, they are also jam packed with nutrients and fiber. They fill you up quickly and keep your digestive system clear which makes you feel so much better.

    Add spices or peppers to it to give it more flavor. Broccoli with a sprinkling of turmeric has been proven to keep prostate cancer at bay as well as help you lose weight.

- **Organic Lean Meats**

    Lean meats contain all of the protein you need without the fat levels but, if you are looking to lose weight, go for organic meats. With normal meats, the animals are pumped full of growth hormones, antibiotics and other nasty things which all end up in what you get on your plate and can slow down your weight loss.

    Organic meat do not contain any more nutrients than normal meat but this is a case of what it doesn't contain that makes it better. If organic is not n supply, look for grass-fed or all-natural brands.

- **Cantaloupe Melon**

    There are those who say that eating a cantaloupe burns off more calories than it contains but that is still up for debate. Whatever the outcome, it is a great food for helping to lose weight because, while it is sweet, it is low in calories, contains fiber and helps keep you moving.

It is good on its own, in a fruit salad or even in a smoothie with other fruits and vegetables. Cantaloupe melon can also help to keep your skin looking great.

- **Spinach**

Spinach is so often left lying on the plate but it is a fantastic food for health and weight loss. It is full of antioxidants, vitamins and minerals and is good to eat in a number of ways. Cook it, eat it raw in a salad, however you want. It adds bulk without adding calories. Try to go for organic and buy in bulk if you buy fresh because you can freeze it for a later date.

- **Green Tea**

Green tea is full of antioxidants and can help you to burn off fat. This is because green tea contains catechins, which help your body to start burning off more calories and well as fat. It isn't processed like so many other teas are and is packed with antioxidants and phytonutrients that make it one of the superstar super foods.

- **Cinnamon**

Cinnamon is one of the most powerful spices and is no longer just used for cooking. Instead, you can get the benefits from cinnamon by adding a teaspoon a day into your diet. It works by regulating your blood sugar levels, which also plays a big part in the way you are feeling throughout the day.

Low blood sugar levels are indicated by a sluggish heavy feeling. Keeping your sugar levels even can also help to stop cravings. One good way is to have a drink of honey and cinnamon in hot water every day.

- **Asparagus**

Asparagus plays a big role in weight loss with lots of different benefits and each benefit plays a specific role in weight loss.

Asparagus helps to eliminate toxins from the body, helps with the digestion process and leaves the good bacteria thriving in your gut. It also has loads of vitamins, minerals and antioxidants. It tastes nice and can also be boosted with spices and seasonings.

- **Avocado**

Avocado is a great slimming aid and contain loads of healthy fats. They were avoided for a long time because of that fat content, at a time when fat was given the label of being evil but we now know that not all fats are bad and that god fats can help to burn fat.

Add avocado to salads, sandwiches, eat them as they are or make your own guacamole with them.

- **Peanut Butter**

  Peanut butter contains good fats that help to burn fat but do go for organic peanut butter as it doesn't contain any of them extra salt and sugar and tat standard peanut butter contains.

  It can be eaten as part of a smoothie or a piece of celery dipped in peanut butter makes a great filling snack. You can also have almond butter but it is more expensive.

- **Salmon**

  Salmon, like other fish, contains a high level of omega 3 and this is one thing that is sorely lacking in many diets today. It may be classed as a fatty fish but it is not high in saturated fats, which are the bad fats and the omega 3 content makes it better than anything else.

  You would need to add this in gradually to see how your body takes to it so start with once a week. If you get on with it, increase that and look around for some great tasting salmon recipes.

- **Apple Cider Vinegar**

  Go for raw organic apple cider vinegar because it contains enzymes that help your digestive system and can help with weight loss over time. The recommended way is to add it to filtered or distilled water and drink it before you eat; this helps your food to be properly digested so that your body gets all the goodness from the nutrients instead of wasting them. It can also help suppress the appetite so drink it if you find yourself hungry between meals.

- **Greek Yoghurt**

Greek yoghurt is healthier than any other yoghurt because it is full of proteins and has a lower sugar content than normal yoghurt.

You don't have to use it as a substitute for normal yoghurt though; you can use it in place of sour cream, cutting down fat and calories and you can also experiment with baking, using it in place of other fats and oils. This could take a bit of trial and error to get it right though.

- **Olive Oil**

Olive oil is a much healthier oil than vegetable or seed oils and it can be used in a variety of ways. Not only can you add it to salads, either on its own or as part of a salad dressing, you can also use it for cooking in.

- **Blueberries**

Blueberries are excellent for fat loss, not just weight. They help to break down sugars and fats in the body as well as tasting amazing. You can use them to add flavor to any meal and they also go well with other fruits – just skip the cream and sugar! Add them to yoghurt or oatmeal for a tasty breakfast or snack.

- **Turkey Breast**

Turkey breast is good for those moments when you are hungry and feel as though you are going to cave in. It is a good source of lean protein and is popular on low or no carb diets. It is a god meat to eat if you are strength training and building up muscle, as well as being able to boost your metabolism.

- **Flax Seeds**

Flax seed can be sprinkled on just about anything you want and it is a better option than sugar. It contains healthy doses of fiber, omega 3 and helps to keep you feeling fuller for longer. The essential fatty acids contained in flax seed helps to boost metabolism and lower bad cholesterol levels.

- **Use Fresh and Organic**

Use fresh ingredients wherever possible and stick to organic. Processed foods are lower in antioxidants and have little weight loss power left in them. Organic foods are best because they don't contain the chemicals and have not been genetically modified.

You can make soups and smoothies out of some of the ingredients on this list and this is a great way to get the benefits without eating a plate of raw food.

Soup is excellent for weight loss and is helps with the digestion process and you can put lots of different foods together in the same soup for a real fat busting meal that is packed full of vitamins.

You can have the soup as a starter or as a meal on its own. It is also much easier to digest than some foods.

Others who are considering purchasing this book would love to know what you think. If you could spare a few seconds, they would greatly appreciate reading an honest review from you. Simply visit the page on Amazon.com.

20 Tasty Super Food Smoothies and Soup Recipes

The following recipes all contain superfoods and are another alternative as a way of making sure that you get all you need in your diet. With the smoothies, simply add all the ingredients to your blender, whiz them up and enjoy!

Peanut Butter Power Shake

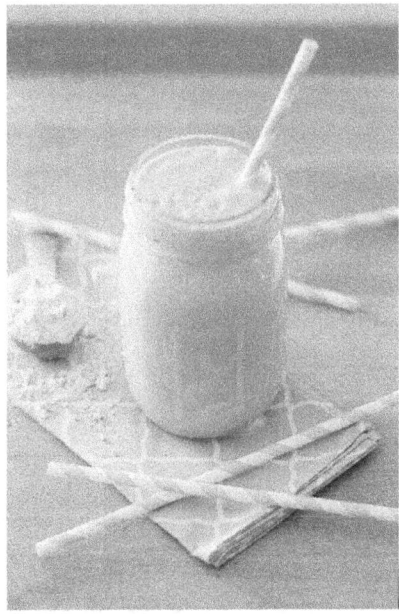

- 1 scoop of whey protein powder, chocolate flavored
- 1 tbsp. organic or natural peanut butter
- ½ banana
- 1 cup of almond milk
- Ice cubes

Dark Chocolate Shake

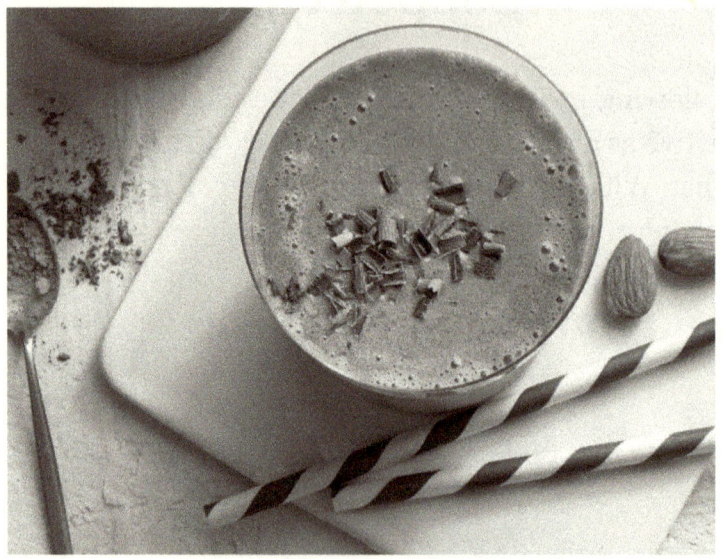

- 1 scoop whey protein, chocolate flavored
- 1 cup almond milk
- 2 ½ tbsp. cacao powder
- 2 ice cubes

CHIA Green Smoothie

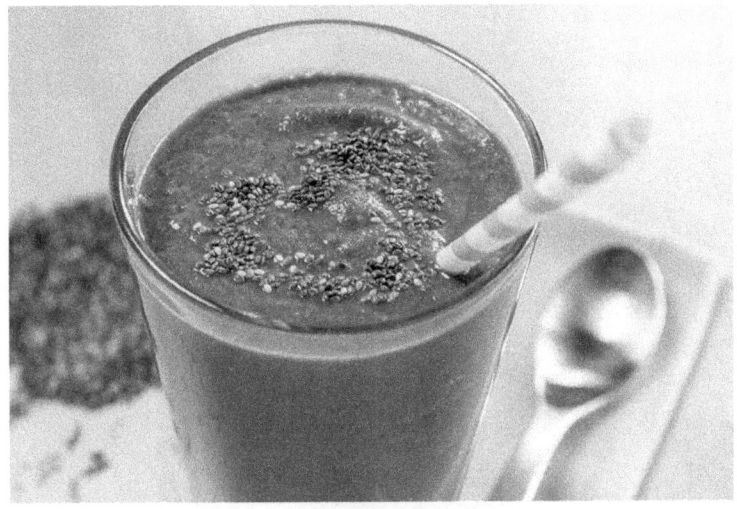

- 1 scoop whey protein vanilla
- 1 tbsp. chia seeds
- 1 cup spinach
- 1 cup almond milk
- 1 banana
- water/ice

The Winter Mint Chocolate Shake

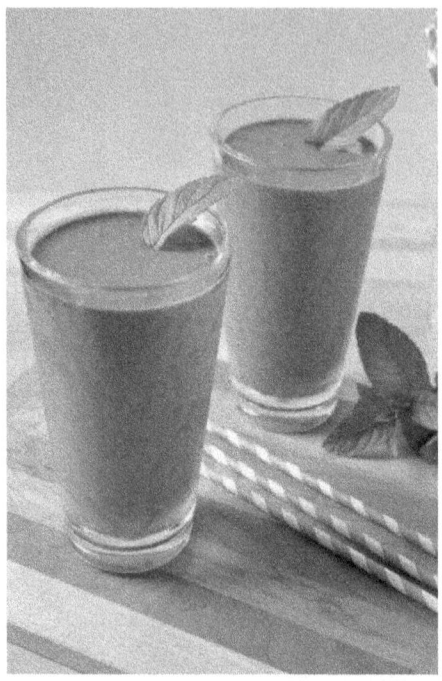

- 1 scoop whey protein, chocolate or chocolate mint
- 1 cup almond milk
- 1/2 cup arctic zero mint chocolate
- 1 drop peppermint extract
- 2 ice cubes

Green Spinach-Apple-Mango Yogurt Smoothie

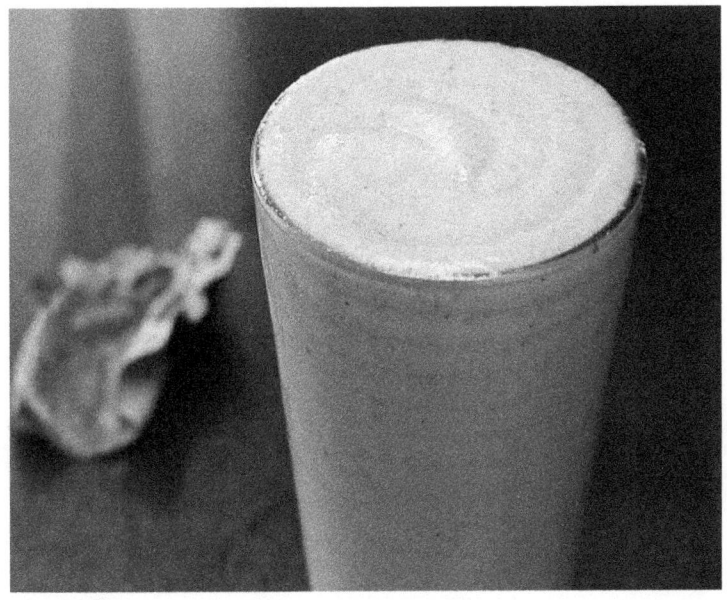

- 3/4 cup plain 0% Greek yogurt
- 1/2 bunch spinach
- 1 apple
- 1/2 cup mango chunks
- 1 cup ice/water

Anti-Aging Kiwi-Blueberry Smoothie

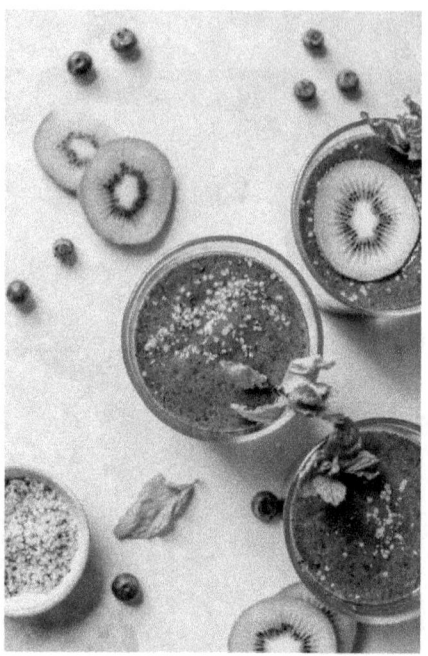

- 1/2 scoop whey protein, vanilla
- 1/2 cup 0% plain Greek yogurt
- 1 cup flax milk
- 2 kiwi
- 1/2 cup blueberries
- 2 ice cubes

Berry Banana Smoothie

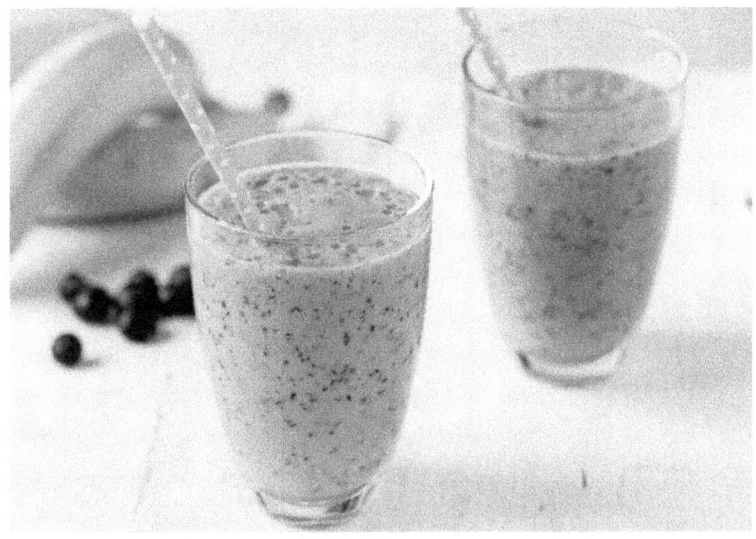

- 1 scoop whey protein, vanilla
- 1 cup flax milk
- 1/2 cup blackberries
- 1/2 banana
- 1/2 cup raspberries
- 1/2 cup strawberries
- 2 ice cubes

Peach-Mango Yogurt Smoothie

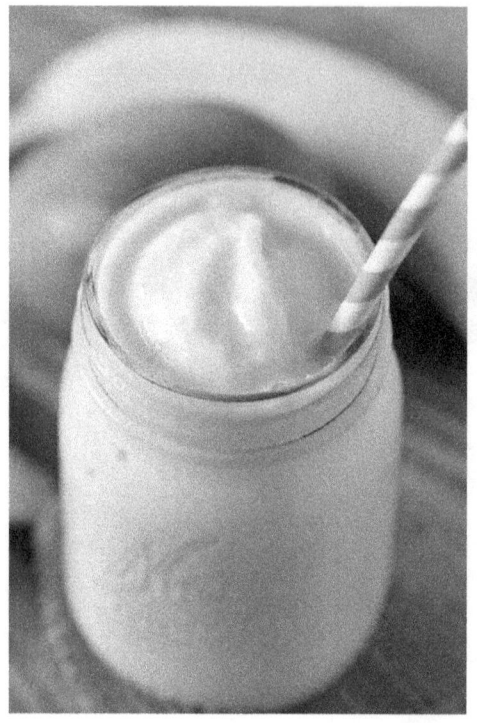

- 1 Cup plain 0% Greek yogurt
- 1 peach
- 1 cup mango chunks
- 1/4 tsp. cinnamon
- 1 cup ice

The Lean Muscle Mochaccino

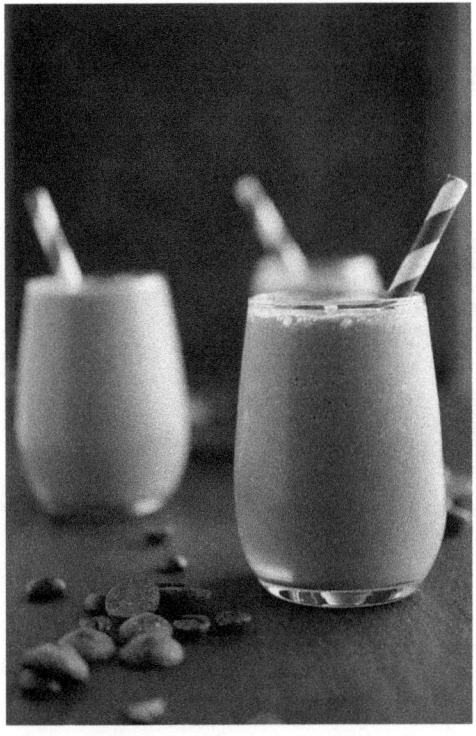

- 1 scoop whey protein, mocha cappuccino
- 1.5 cups flax milk
- 2.5 tbsp. cacao powder
- 2 ice cubes

Orange Creamsicle Smoothie

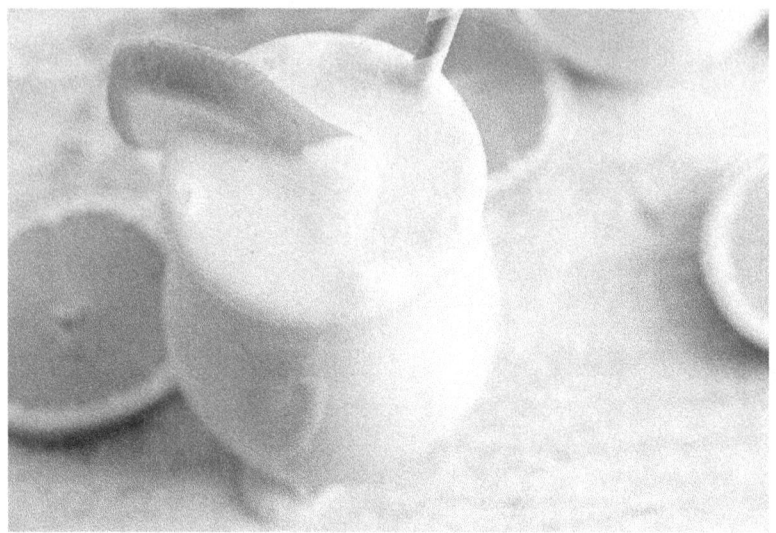

- 1 scoop whey protein, orange creamsicle
- 1 medium orange
- 1 cup almond milk
- 1/2 cup orange juice
- 1 cup water/ice

Liquid Breakfast Smoothie

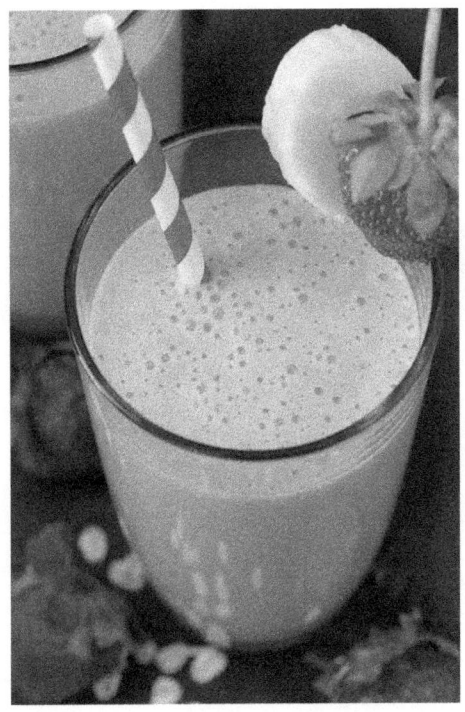

- 3/4 cup plain 0% Greek yogurt
- 1/2 banana
- 1/4 cup rolled oats
- 1 cup strawberries
- 1 cup water/Ice

Banana Nut Shake

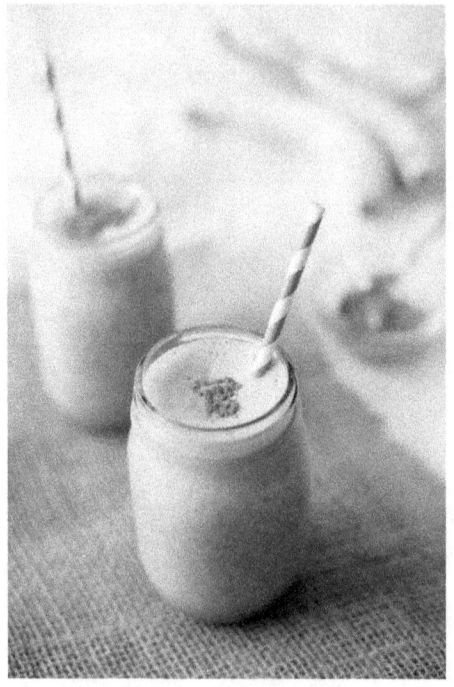

- 1 scoop vanilla whey protein
- 1 cup almond milk
- 1 large banana
- 3 tbsp. organic peanut butter
- water/ice

Strawberry Shortcake Smoothie

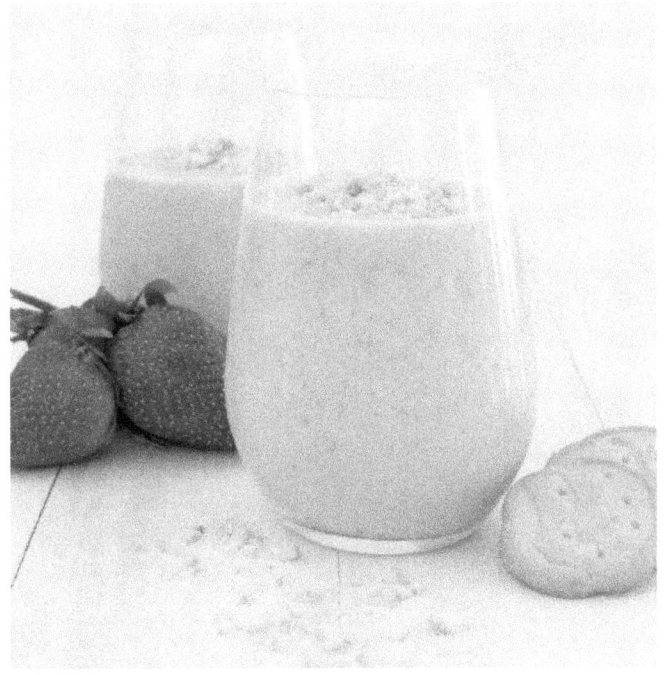

- 3/4 cup plain 0% Greek yogurt
- 1 cup strawberries
- 1/2 cup rolled oats
- 1 tsp vanilla extract
- water/ice

Mango Pineapple Shake

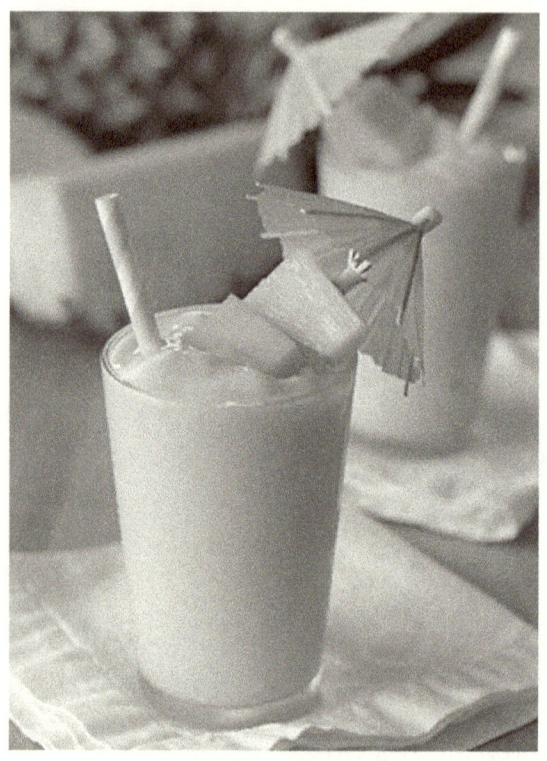

- 1 scoop vanilla whey protein
- 1/2 cup mango chunks
- 1/2 cup pineapple chunks
- 1 cup almond Milk

Creamy Chocolate Avocado Smoothie

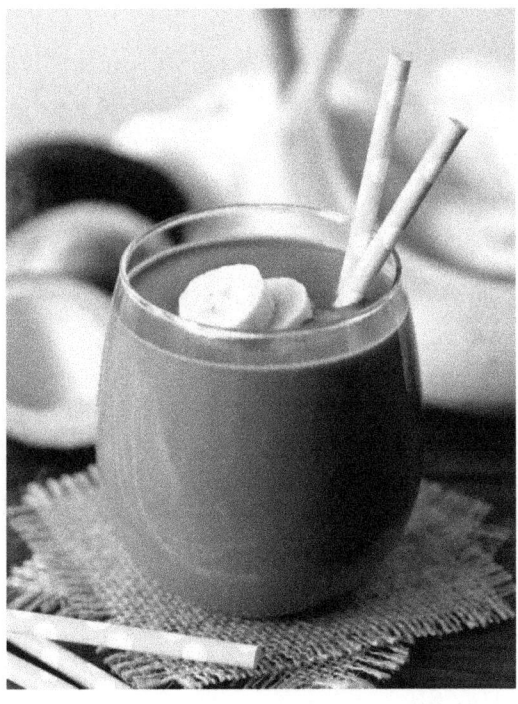

- 1 scoop chocolate whey protein
- 1/2 small avocado
- 3/4 banana
- 1 1/2 cup ice/Water

Green Superfood Soup

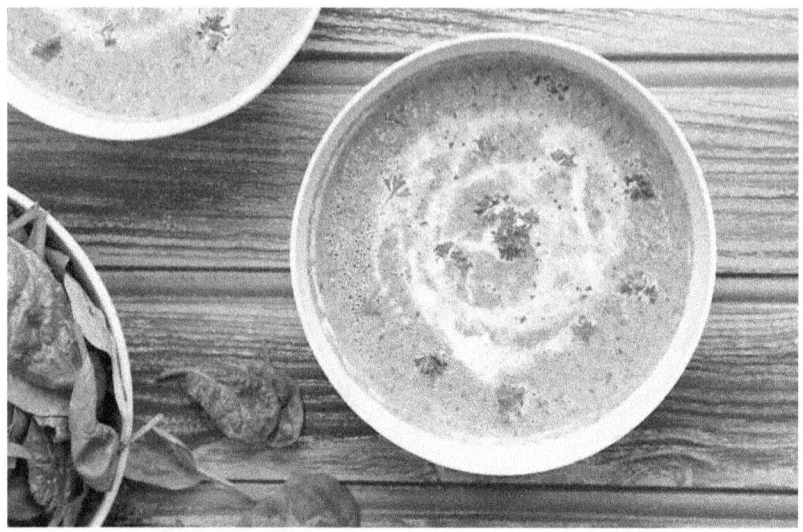

Ingredients

- 185 g broccoli
- 2 leeks sliced
- 1 onion roughly diced
- ½ teaspoon garlic oil or minced garlic
- 1 cup green split peas – soaked for 1 hour, rinsed
- 310 g medium cauliflower
- 9-10 g dry wakame seaweed – soaked for 10 min, roughly chopped
- 80 g kale – roughly chopped
- ½ cup stock
- pinch sea salt
- pepper
- ¼ tsp thyme
- enough water to cover

- Oil for cooking
- Coconut cream

Instructions

1. Heat up the oil in a large pan. Cook the onions and leeks until they are brown.

2. Add all other ingredients, add the stock and enough water to cover the vegetables.

3. Simmer for about 1 hour over a low heat, or until the split peas are soft.

4. Blend in the blender to make a thick soup.

5. Add in some coconut cream and water to bring it to the consistency you like. Season with salt and pepper.

Carrot and Turmeric Soup

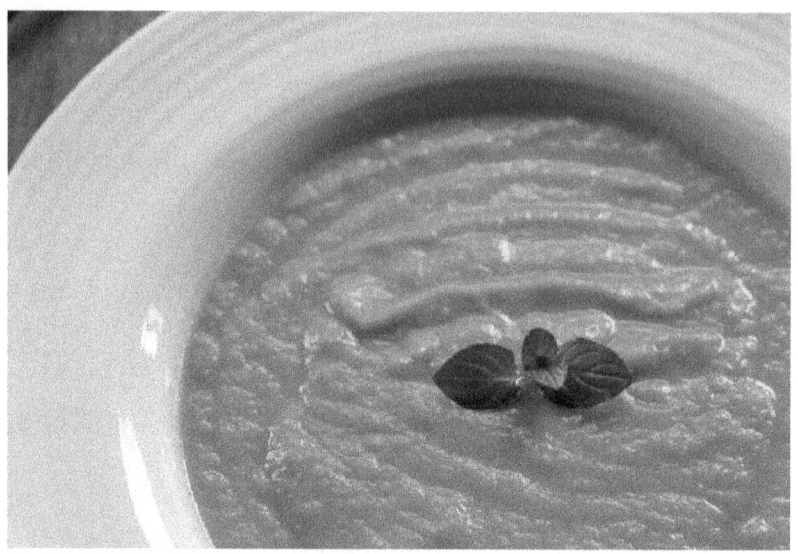

Ingredients

- 500 g carrots
- 2 garlic cloves
- 1 onion, white
- 1 tbsp. coconut oil
- 2 tsp turmeric
- 1 tbsp. fresh ginger
- 400 ml stock
- 150 ml water
- Salt and pepper
- 1 lime

Instructions

1. Chop the carrots into pieces about an inch in size and peel the garlic; set aside. Cut the onion into small bits and fry over a medium heat with a pinch of salt and 1 tbsp. oil.

2. Add the ginger and turmeric and cook for 30 seconds, stirring. Crush the garlic and add it in, stir and add the carrots. Roast for a few minutes before adding the stock.

3. Use a blender to blend the soup until smooth – add more water if needed. Add another inch of salt, pepper and squeeze the juice in from the lime.

Dairy-Free Creamy Avocado Soup

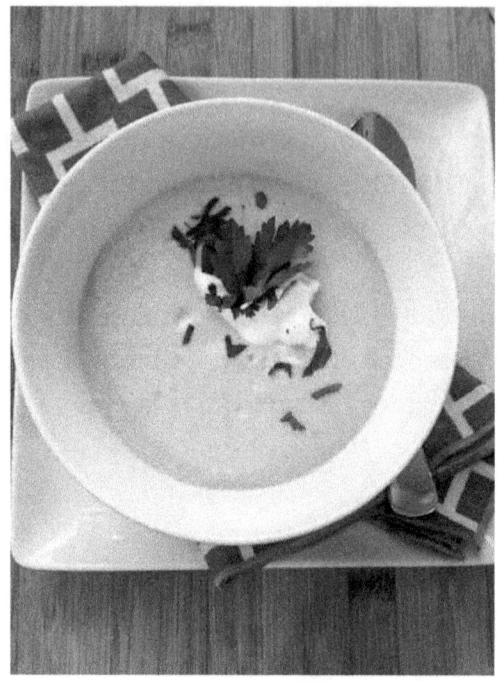

Ingredients

- 3 ripe avocado, peeled, pitted and chopped
- 2 cups plain dairy-free yogurt
- 1/3 cup cashews
- 1/3 cup finely chopped fresh cilantro
- 1/3 cup vidalia onion, chopped
- 1 Tbsp. white balsamic vinegar
- 1 cup green tea, brewed and chilled
- 1 tsp. sea salt
- ¼ tsp. freshly ground white pepper
- 2 chives, finely chopped

Instructions

1. Blend the avocado, yoghurt, cilantro, almonds, onion, vinegar, green tea, pepper and sea salt until smooth.

2. Transfer into a bowl and cover; refrigerate for 2 hours. Serve chilled and garnished with chopped chives.

Spicy Chicken and Quinoa Soup

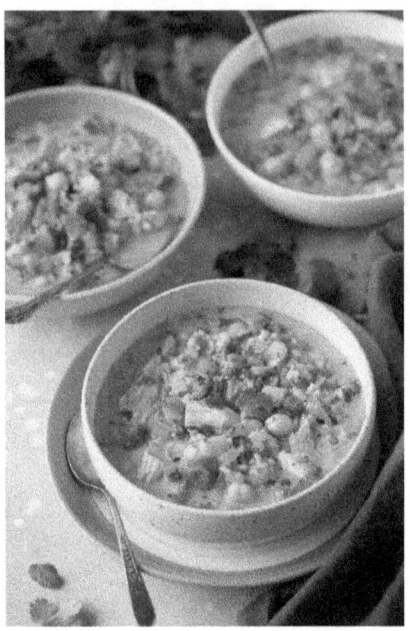

Ingredients

- 2 tbsp. extra virgin olive oil
- 1 cup diced onion
- 2 garlic cloves, chopped
- 2 tomatoes, peeled and diced
- 2 carrots, peeled and chopped
- 1 tsp of paprika
- 2 tsp of cumin
- 2 cups of white meat from 2 baked skinless and shredded organic chicken breasts
- 2 cups of filtered water
- 4 cups low sodium organic chicken broth
- 2 cups of fresh or frozen peas

- 2 cups cooked quinoa
- 4 tbsp. finely chopped parsley
- 3 tbsp. finely chopped cilantro
- 1 tsp kosher salt
- Freshly ground black pepper

Instructions

1. Heat up the olive oil in a large soup pot. Add the onions, garlic and sauté until translucent, about 5 minutes.

2. Add the tomato, carrots, cumin and pepper, cook for a father 5 minutes, stirring. Add the water and broth, turn the heat up to high and bring to a boil.

3. Add the peas, quinoa, herbs and chicken, season with salt and pepper. Reduce heat and simmer for 25 minutes. Serve hot with a diced avocado.

To Bake Chicken Breasts

1. Preheat the oven to 350° F. Rub olive oil over the chicken and season with salt and pepper.

2. Place in a foil lined baking sheet, skin side up and bake for 40 to 45 minutes.

3. Remove and allow it to cool off before taking the skin off and shredding it.

Slow Cooker Superfood Soup

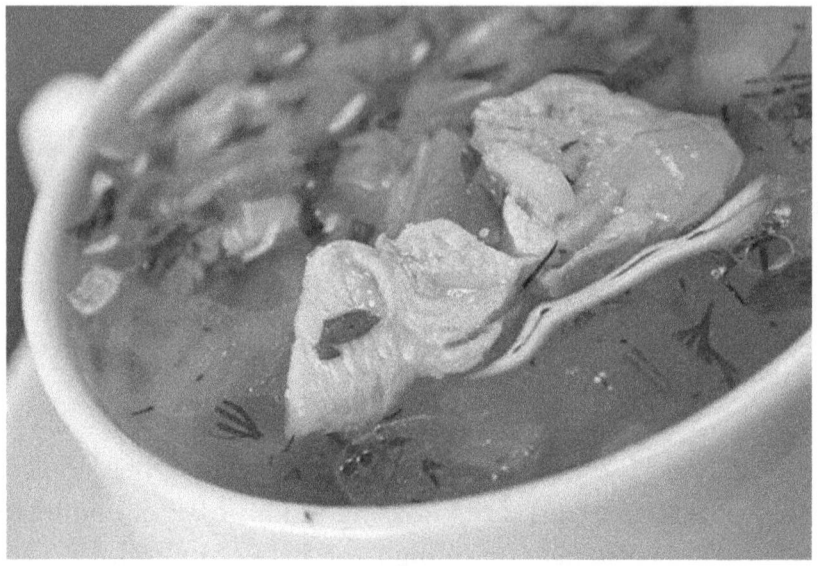

Ingredients

- 2 cups sliced carrots
- 1 large sweet potato, cut into 1/2" cubes
- 1 cup fresh or frozen green beans
- 1/2 cup fresh cilantro, chopped
- 1 small onion, diced
- 1 clove garlic, minced
- 2 (15 ounce) cans black beans, drained and rinsed
- 1/2 teaspoon crushed red pepper flakes
- 1/2 teaspoon black pepper
- 1 teaspoon chili powder
- 1 teaspoon cumin
- Kosher or sea salt to taste

- 2 cups vegetable juice (I used R.W. Knudsen, Organic Very Veggie Juice, no sugar added)
- 2 cups vegetable broth, low-sodium

Instructions

1. Mix all the ingredients together in your slow cooker, cover and cook it for about 6-8 hours on low, or until the vegetables have gone tender. If you want, you can add in a tbsp. of low fat cheddar cheese

2. You can sauté onion in 1 tbsp. olive oil for 5 minutes and then add the garlic and sauté for a further 1 minute before adding them to the slow cooker.

3. You can also add in 2 cups of coarsely chopped kale about 5 minutes before the end of cooking

I hope you have learned something from this book so far and would greatly appreciate it if you could leave an honest review on Amazon.com.

8 Reasons Why You Are Not Losing Body Fat

Collectively, we spend years of our lives trying to shed those extra pounds of body fat but have little to no success.

We go on diet after diet, our weight yo-yoing up and down and we ride on a rollercoaster that has way too much roll in it. We try to shed the fat when we are motivated but still fall apart when we see a plate of fresh warm cookies.

Unfortunately, this is why so many New Year's resolutions wind up discarded and gym memberships get ignored. While we might have a common goal in mind, losing fat, it is not an easy thing to achieve satisfactorily.

If you have been playing the same game and haven't yet succeeded, you are more than likely making a couple of mistakes. Below I am going to talk about the 8 most common mistakes that people make when they are trying to lose fat:

Mistake Number 1 – You are eating too much

This might seem like an obvious on but so many people seriously do not know how many calories they are eating. A salad might seem like a low-calorie option but you may actually be munching your way through 600 calories.

Salad dressings, sauces, ketchups and oils are all loaded with calories that you don't always see or think about, especially if you are not a regular cook at home.

We are always told to eat less calories than we are burning but this simplifies matters too much. This would work if you, for example, ate 1500 calories worth of cheesecake every day and burned 2000 calories. But, the one thing the human body can't do is be a calculator. What matters is not how many calories but the type of calories you are eating.

If you eat a diet that is made up of carbohydrates only, you won't burn any fat, whereas if you eat less of the carbs and more protein, fat and the right carbs, you are on to a winning combination for burning fat and building up muscle.

Most people find that a ratio of 40% carbs, 40% protein and 20% fat works perfectly to burn off that fat. However, that may not work for all so you will need to do your research and work out what is best for you.

Some people have to reduce their carb limit even lower to be successful but, if you have to do that, boost up your good fat intake to allow your body an alternative source of energy to burn.

Mistake Number 2 – You are not eating enough protein

Protein isn't just for building and repairing your muscle tissue. Recent studies have showed that, on two groups of women who were overweight, both of whom consumed the same number of calories per day, the group that consumed 128 g protein every day lost more weight than the group who consumed just 68 g protein per day.

Protein makes you feel fuller for much longer and stops you from grazing throughout the day and from eating too much at your main meals. A high protein diet can also affect the glucose levels, blood lipids and muscle to fat ratio in the body in a positive manner.

Protein is an excellent fat loss macro but you will not see instant results by adding protein shakes to your diet. Fat burning is not instant; it takes dedication and consistently following the meal plan to make a difference. What you can do is add high protein foods to your meals and cut down on the bad carbs foods – you will see the results in time.

Mistake Number 3 – You are drinking too much

You really only need to drink water. You can have tea or coffees, occasionally milk but stop the stream of sugar-filled drinks. All they are doing is undoing the good work the rest of your food is doing. One pumpkin spice latte can contain over 300 calories, and that is just in one drink! That is not doing your body any good at all – all you are doing is making your fat loss goas harder to attain.

Alcohol is also a bad call. While a beer or a glass of wine every now and again isn't going to make much difference, you must stop the binging at weekends.

Alcohol is high in calories, these are stored by your body as fat, and it also causes an impairment to your judgment. Instead of eating a good healthy choice, the booze will tell you that a big pate of cheesy chips is just the right thing to eat.

Mistake Number 4 – You think that healthy foods have no calories

Everything has calories in it, regardless of how healthy it is. If you eat too much, you will struggle to shed the fat. Of course, you need to eat whole foods but eating too much organic peanut butter is still overeating whichever you look at it.

Two examples of healthy foods that are significantly high in calories are seeds and nuts. They contain micronutrients, omega 3 and phytogens that are absolutely wonderful for your health but are excessively high in calories. Don't avoid them; just stick to eating a small handful at a time.

Mistake Number 5 – Your training regime is not intensive enough

While it is important for complete beginners to start off slowly, you should gradually up your game, as you become more and more used to the gym machines, weights and the actual exercise itself.

Start to push yourself harder and harder – if you get comfortable doing your training, your weight loss will simply plateau. If you are not breaking a sweat through your exercise, you are not working out hard enough. If you are not sweating, you are not burning fat and your heart rate is not working to your benefit.

If you are looking to burn fat, you need to create an extreme energy demand so that your body is able to change. Lifting the same old weights time and time again will not help you to burn fat and you won't be gaining any real benefits from your physical activity.

Mistake Number 6 – You are doing too much low intensity cardio training

Ok, so I just told you to up the intensity of your workout and now I'm telling you off for doing too much of something that isn't intensive. Cardio is not a form of resistance training. It is a completely different type of fitness and a two-hour slog on the treadmill is not going to give you the results that an hour of heavy lifting will.

If you want your cardio to work, do full body workouts that include a short rest period. By using your whole body and taking shorter breaks, your cardiovascular system and your muscular system are being challenged.

Mistake Number 7 – You are stressed out

Stress is one of the biggest and most silent killers. Stress causes your body to produce cortisol in levels way beyond what is normal. This can be responsible to an increase in fat storage in the body and many other negative consequences. Even if your diet and your training regime are spot-on, if you re stressed, you will not achieve your goals.

The key is to relax and, although that is easier said than done, if you can learn some deep breathing, meditation, or yoga and incorporate it every day in your diet, you will see a significant change in your overall health and in your physique

Mistake 8 – You are not sleeping enough

Sleep deprivation also raises cortisol levels and, when you are lacking in sleep; your insulin sensitivity is also reduced. Together, these two problems are not good news for anyone who wants to burn fat.

Sleep is a priority in your life. You cannot possibly party all night and expect to function well the next day. Aim for 8 hours of good sleep every single night.

Don't drink alcohol, don't use your tablet, mobile phone or watch TV for at least an hour before you go to bed, eliminate caffeine in the evenings and give yourself time to relax in the evenings.

Don't forget to share your thoughts on this book by leaving a review on Amazon.com. It takes just a few seconds.

Weight Loss is HARD!

Discover How to Make It EASIER to Lose Weight & Keep It OFF Forever (This Is The ONLY Book You NEED to Read)

For this month only, you can get Sarah's best-selling & most popular guide absolutely free – *The #1 Weight Loss Guide*.

Get Your FREE Copy Here:
TopFitnessAdvice.com/Freebie

It's time to stop struggling with your weight loss efforts that don't seem to work.

Discover how you can start seeing real results by next week (without changing much in your life). With this guide, readers were able to significantly improve their weight loss results. So, it's highly recommended that you get this guide, especially while it's free!

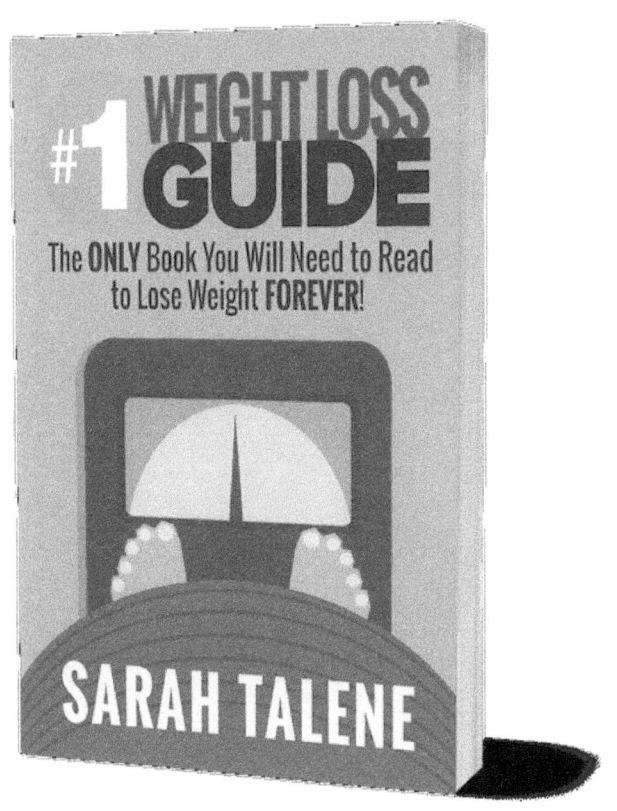

Get Your FREE Copy Here:
TopFitnessAdvice.com/Freebie

Conclusion

Now, that wasn't so hard, was it?

It's amazing how easily we can adjust to healthy eating. It's also amazing how quickly our bodies start repairing themselves once they get the nutrition they need.

I hope that you have started incorporating these tips into your daily life already.

If not, I urge you to start doing so without delay. In just a week, you will start to feel like a new person – your mind becomes clearer, you are less sluggish and you crave less junk food.

After just two or three weeks, you will never want to go back to eating as you did before.

And that is where this plan is different – it is not a diet that is unsustainable. It is an adjustment in the way you eat that is easy to stick to.

Good eating should never feel like a hardship. I hope that this is something that this plan has taught you.

I wish you all the best with the new you!

Enjoying this book?

Check out my other best sellers!

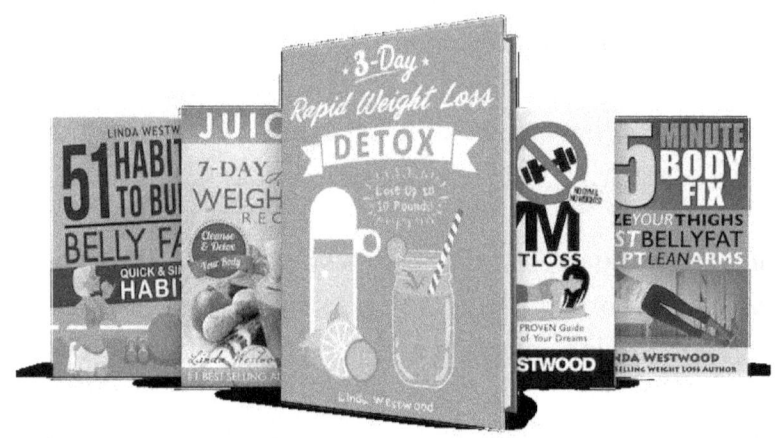

Get your next book on sale here:

TopFitnessAdvice.com/go/books

Final Words

I would like to thank you for purchasing my book and I hope I have been able to help you and educate you on something new.

If you have enjoyed this book and would like to share your positive thoughts, could you please take 30 seconds of your time to go back and give me a review on my Amazon book page.

I greatly appreciate seeing these reviews because it helps me share my hard work.

You can leave me a review on Amazon.com.

Again, thank you and I wish you all the best!

www.ingramcontent.com/pod-product-compliance
Lightning Source LLC
Chambersburg PA
CBHW031200020426
42333CB00013B/765